BODY WISDOM JOURNAL

BODY WISDOM JOURNAL

40 Days to Heal & Listen to Your Body's Intuition

Alegra Loewenstein

For ordering information or special discounts for bulk pricing, please contact alegra@healthyfamilyharmony.com

First Edition: 2018

Cover Design and Formatting by: Allysa Milad

Author Photos by: Anna Day Mona

ISBN-13: 978-1986839754

ISBN-10: 1986839753

Printed in the United States of America

TABLE OF CONTENTS

WHAT IS BODY WISDOM?

Body wisdom is a very simple concept; it's the idea that our bodies have information that isn't available to us strictly through our minds. It is also the ability to know your own body, be the expert of your own body, and perhaps most importantly, love and trust your own body.

We have all heard the phrase "listen to your body," but it's not always easy to know how to do so. This journal is designed to give you daily practices to actually help you listen to your body, and to help you practice listening to your body so that it becomes easy and natural to do!

WHY WE NEED BODY WISDOM

Our modern world is a busy, hectic place. We are often too busy to pay attention to our bodies. We are often disconnected by how we look at and approach our health. We are not taught to trust our own bodies; we are taught to trust the experts, not ask questions, and treat isolated problems.

While this is changing to some extent, and larger health care facilities are beginning to offer holistic approaches to health, change is slow. We can speed this process along by connecting with our body, building up our own intuition, and learning to communicate with our own bodies in a meaningful way. This journal will help you collaborate with your medical care provider, and it will also help you build up the confidence and personal knowledge of your own body to challenge the medical system when it isn't actually serving you as a patient. Your doctor is the expert on the ailment, but you are the expert on your own experience.

BODY WISDOM AND BODY ESTEEM

We also need to come to terms with low body esteem, which is an epidemic in this country. Our media has ruined our ability to feel good about our own bodies. Our media has inundated us with twisted images and messages about what we need to look like to be pretty enough, happy enough, and good enough. It is a toxic formula that poisons our minds, starting almost from infancy. Despite progress over the generations for women's rights, the influence of our own perception has still been swayed simply by the images we are repeatedly exposed to on the TV, on social media, even in the check-out line. Our loved ones pick up these messages, and, despite their best intentions, they often reinforce them. Women have it worse, but sadly the messages men receive are almost catching up in their effect on body esteem.

The truth is that our body esteem affects our self-esteem AND our ability to have body wisdom! The good news is that you can create higher body esteem and therefore higher self-esteem. You can also learn to recognize your self-esteem as separate from your body esteem.

Improving your body esteem and self-esteem will also boost your own intuition, which will help you tune into your body wisdom and reinforce all these improvements.

It is a positive feedback cycle that makes you feel better and better! However, you do have to do the work. It might feel like an uphill battle in the beginning, but I promise you that you will come out on top, feeling more amazing than ever before!

Aspects of this journal are designed to make sure you are working to combat the body esteem ruining messages out there. The good news is that it IS possible to turn this around! My client C.L. wrote down several affirmations and hung them on her mirror to start the process of feeling better about herself, and it worked! If she can do it, so can you!

Some additional tips to help improve body esteem:

• Be selective about your media; avoid magazines that showcase unrealistic women's bodies, including gossip magazines, fashion magazines, and all mainstream women's magazines; seek out body affirming content instead. Sadly, it is very hard to find body positive content in most mainstream stores, but you can seek it out and sign up online.

• Use affirmations regularly. There is hard science behind affirmations. The more we see/say/think things, the more easily our mind absorbs them. You can actually change your body esteem and self-esteem with words!

• Get the support you need to make sure you are taking health-aligned action in your life. My clients often struggle to make healthy choices, and a lot of it has to do with feeling misaligned in values and actions or simply suffering low self-esteem or low body esteem that sabotages healthy choices. My program can help turn that around. Invest in yourself to feel your best, whether by signing up for one of my programs or simply by getting a partner or best friend to do a journal with you; you need support to succeed!

HOW TO GET THE MOST OUT
OF THIS JOURNAL

Think Outside the Body

I have gone through times in my life when I took ibuprofen more days than not. I took it for my neck, and then when my neck started feeling better, I took it for headaches. I knew there was a physical, muscular element to this, and that I had to gain strength, which took me several years.

For many years, I suffered neck pain. First, it was intermittent. Then, after my second son was born, it became chronic.

In the beginning, I kept saying that it was caused by imbalanced muscles. This was surely true, at least in part.

However, I was also recovering from the transition to parenthood. This process took much longer to understand and to cope with. I was "shouldering" too much of a burden, and things were out of alignment. I needed more boundaries, more time alone, more enjoyment of the time I did spend with my family. This realization about my neck pain brought me much more balance in my life and ultimately led me to resolve the pain quicker than when I was "just getting physical therapy" – and the physical therapy felt like "just another item on my to do list."

And yet when I started to explore this question deeper, I knew that it was also about carrying a burden that was too great for me to carry. There was no specific event that caused this burden, it was simply that my life required much of me, and I had a hard time fulfilling what was required. Parenthood was part of it.

As it turned out, a lot of that burden I put on myself - and as I began to take it off my own shoulders - no one else had to "pick it up." I just had to set it down. There is no requirement that something "bad" happens in your life before you can simply say that your load is too great. Sometimes we are simply too hard on ourselves, and there is nothing shameful in acknowledging that and beginning to make changes.

My client E. L. battled unwanted weight her whole life. She counted calories and worried about what she should or shouldn't be eating all the time. When she finally recognized that every part of that battle was actually founded on a childhood loss and how it affected her self-esteem (coupled with ignorance from her family regarding young women's bodies and body esteem), she was finally able to begin shedding the weight naturally, without "dieting" anymore. If she could look beyond decades of misperception to see a bigger picture of who she was, so can you!

Try to look beyond the physical and understand the meaning of your physical body in a higher picture way. Here are some tips to guide your process. Feel free to come back to this reference page as you work through the book. Dog-ear it.

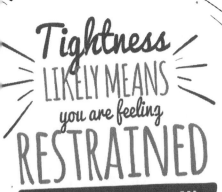

Tightness
LIKELY MEANS
you are feeling
RESTRAINED
IN SOME ASPECT OF YOUR LIFE

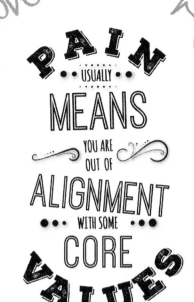

PAIN
...USUALLY...
MEANS
YOU ARE
OUT OF
ALIGNMENT
WITH SOME
CORE
VALUES

BEING
TIRED
USUALLY MEANS NOT
sleeping zᶻᶻ
enough
BUT ON A
BIGGER PICTURE

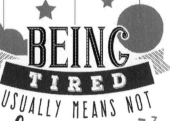

SIGNIFIES
BEING
MAXED
OUT

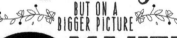

A COMMON CONCERN IN TODAY'S MODERN WORLD
THAT FAILS TO VALUE REST AND NOURISHMENT

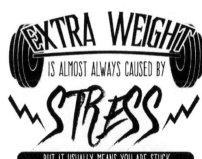

EXTRA WEIGHT
IS ALMOST ALWAYS CAUSED BY
STRESS
BUT IT USUALLY MEANS YOU ARE STUCK
IN OLD
Patterns
>>> THAT RETAIN THE **STRESS** <<<

TUNE INTO YOUR BODY

Sit or lay down in a quiet place for each of the daily prompts. It is important that you are very comfortable and will not be disturbed. It takes time to get to know our bodies, and we tend to not be able to when we are interrupted by the outside world. First thing in the morning or last thing of the day are probably the best times to commit to this practice. It can be hard to fit it in during our hectic days, so tie it in to something you do daily that is associated with quiet... which is probably sleep!

Sometimes you will write. Sometimes you will just sit and listen. The daily questions are mostly about tuning in to your body. If you gain information, you don't always need to write it down, (but of course writing it down helps you continue to process your insights and to more easily remember what you are learning from yourself).

EMPOWER YOUR MIND

However, you must write the affirmations and accomplishments. This stage is the mindset part of the journal, and it is a critical part of your success! By reinforcing positive thoughts about yourself and your body, and by affirming them with daily accomplishments, you begin to feel more aligned with your values and your actions... and this is the secret formula to sustained success!

If you can commit to just doing this portion of the journal daily, you will begin to see amazing progress, and quickly! One of my own coaches literally turned my life around by introducing me to mindset journaling. In just a few weeks I noticed a difference in my attitude about all aspects of my life, and I continue the practice to this day. I often have clients (and other women who have bought my journals) share with me how this simple practice changed their life around. If we can do it, so can you!

So remember...
   • Write an affirmation each day in the first part of the day's prompt.
   • Write an accomplishment each day in the accomplishments part of the day's prompt.

You will also complete four healing rituals throughout the journal. The first day is dedicated to creating a powerful and meaningful affirmation that you can use daily throughout the rest of the journal.

An affirmation in this journal is meant to be a sentence that affirms your personal goals and strengths, and which is written repeatedly to cement it into your brain. This practice helps you believe in yourself and feel empowered even at times when you might otherwise be in doubt. You can also read and speak your affirmations, which are both wonderful ways to further enhance the positive effects your affirmation will have on your mindset. However, for the purpose of this program, you only need to write your affirmation daily.

This journal is created to guide you through the process of learning from your body and healing your body pain – both physical and emotional. Every aspect of this journal was created with intention, based on my training as a health coach, my work with clients, my degree in biology, my lifetime of reading self-help books, and additional research I did on changing mindset, habits, and body perception in order to create this book.

So, on the one hand, I ask you to trust the process and go along with each step. And, on the other hand, this is your journal. Journals are personal, and I believe they represent each of our journeys to understand ourselves and grow... so you can also decide to do things differently if you know another way will serve you better.

In short, trust me... but trust yourself more!!! That is the ultimate goal anyway!

UNDERSTAND YOUR BODY

Part of body wisdom is learning to understand your body, and there are a lot of ways to do that and gain that information. Keep track of your period on this super helpful menstrual chart, broken into 28-day months so you can see if you are on the longer or shorter side of average. Just use a pen, pencil, or highlighter to mark your period – you can mark all the days and see how it varies in length from month to month as well. Heck, you can even chart the heaviness of flow if you want, with a little hump chart on the days you are bleeding heaviest. Feel free to use a little star to mark your ovulation day(s) as well.

Your Monthly Cycle is an important aspect of your body and your mood. Use these quadrants to take notes on the four weeks of your cycle. Of course, not everyone's cycle is exactly 28 days, so just do your best to divide your cycle into approximately quarters, or at least make notes of things that are happening just before/during/after ovulation and menstruation. I suggest taking down notes over more than a month, so don't feel the need to fill up the entire space in one week, but rather jot quick notes as you observe them, and then look for patterns once you have several months' worth.

NOTE IF YOU HAVE NO PERIOD

You can use the quadrants to take notes on an external cycle in your life – a pattern at work, your partner's monthly cycle, moving through the week, or some other pattern you think of. The point is to observe how your body reacts through a cycle to see if you can understand it and use its natural tendencies to your advantage, and of course take care of your body as best you can.

WOMEN: CHARTING YOUR CYCLE

DECEMBER	NOVEMBER	OCTOBER	SEPTEMBER	AUGUST	JULY	JUNE	MAY	APRIL	MARCH	FEBRUARY	JANUARY
29	1	29	1	29	1	29	1	29	1	29	1
30	2	30	2	30	2	30	2	30	2	30	2
31	3	31	3	31	3		3	31	3	31	3
	4		4		4		4		4		4
	5		5		5		5		5		5
	6		6		6		6		6		6
	7		7		7		7		7		7
	8		8		8		8		8		8
	9		9		9		9		9		9
	10		10		10		10		10		10
	11		11		11		11		11		11
	12		12		12		12		12		12
	13		13		13		13		13		13
	14		14		14		14		14		14
	15		15		15		15		15		15
	16		16		16		16		16		16
	17		17		17		17		17		17
	18		18		18		18		18		18
	19		19		19		19		19		19
	20		20		20		20		20		20
	21		21		21		21		21		21
	22		22		22		22		22		22
	23		23		23		23		23		23
	24		24		24		24		24		24
	25		25		25		25		25		25
	26		26		26		26		26		26
	27		27		27		27		27		27
	28		28		28		28		28		28

WEEK 1: MENSTRUATION

DATE	OBSERVATION/NOTES
_____	_____
	_____
_____	_____
	_____
_____	_____
	_____
_____	_____
	_____
_____	_____
	_____

PATTERNS I'VE NOTICED

WEEK 2: INCREASING ENERGY

DATE

OBSERVATION/NOTES

_____   _____

_____

_____   _____

_____

_____   _____

_____

_____   _____

_____

_____   _____

_____

PATTERNS I'VE NOTICED

WEEK 3: OVULATION

DATE	OBSERVATION/NOTES
_____	_____
_____	_____
_____	_____
_____	_____
_____	_____

PATTERNS I'VE NOTICED

WEEK 4: SLOWING DOWN

DATE	OBSERVATION/NOTES
_____	_____
	_____
_____	_____
	_____
_____	_____
	_____
_____	_____
	_____
_____	_____
	_____

PATTERNS I'VE NOTICED

Week 1: *Menstruation*
You may find you are tired in this week. This is normal. Your body is cleansing and processing an entire uterine lining. Give it a break; if you are tired, take a nap. It can be powerful to see that you need naps this one week AND allow yourself to have them, and you will likely feel better all month.

Week 2: *Increasing energy*
Women often begin to feel better and more energized this week. Take notes on how this may be true for you, perhaps more social or productive. You can utilize this. Some women ovulate this week.

Week 3: *Ovulation*
This may be a time of high energy or continuing to feel what you felt in week 2. Take note so you can have this awareness about yourself and your cycle. By the way, do you know how to tell if you are ovulating? It is often, but not always, about halfway through your cycle. Many of us get a super slimy, sometimes sticky wad of gooey discharge on that day that looks and feels like egg white... very often it comes out when you poo, so check the paper, 'kay? (I know, I know... well, it IS a Body Wisdom book, we do have to talk about that amazing body!) Some women also get a one-time cramp around that time, and some women get super horny! Being knowledgeable about your body isn't just for people trying to get pregnant, though having the knowledge already might help if or when that time comes.

Week 4: *Slowing Down*

You may find heightened physical or emotional sensitivity during the week before menstruation. Yes, this is often called PMS and treated as a useless pain in the ass (or worse by some people), but it's actually really useful information! You are sensitive at this time! Your "PMS" may be a sign that your life isn't aligned with what your body needs, but you only feel it at this more sensitive point in your cycle. You may be more susceptible to pain or illness. Slow down and take care of yourself. Some women ovulate this week.

DAY 1
HEALING RITUAL

Today you begin a journey of healing. You might complete it in 40 days, or you might take breaks and detours and do it in bits and pieces. However you do it is fine. Take a deep breath right now. Let go of any expectations you have. Let go of any "shoulds" or "must-do's. Let this process unfold in a loving, healing, and gentle way.

Let's start this journey by setting your intention for the journal. Spend 5 minutes and write down all things you WANT to gain from this journal. Write down all the things you want to FEEL about and in your body. Write down all the things you want to THINK to yourself when you look in the mirror. Don't doubt or second guess yourself, just write all the dreams and hopes you have for this process.

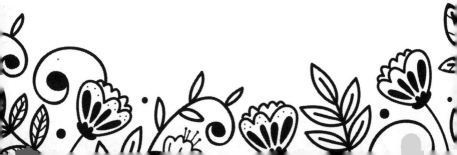

Now, go back through and circle and put stars and exclamation points. Mark it up; get in touch with the ones that feel really important. If they trigger doubt, fear, or an inner eye roll, put them in parentheses or add a question mark. But don't scratch them out. We are staying open to possibilities here.

Finally… pick one. If one feels too hard, pick two or three to start with, knowing that you will feel them out and choose one. This is your intention for the journal. Write this into an affirmation that starts with "I" (or similar) and is in present tense. Use this space to refine it.

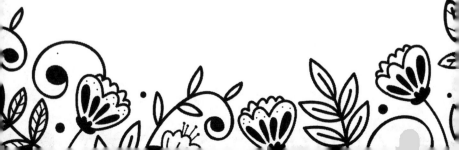

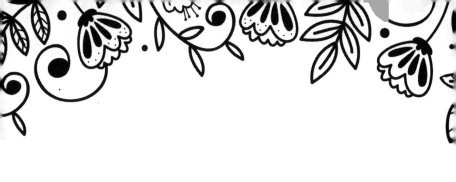

Examples:

     I am proud of who I am.

     My soul shines every day.

     I am healthy.

     I love to smile.

     I am awesome!

     I love my life.

     I am safe.

Pick one you are really excited about, because I want you to write the same affirmation every day for the next 40 days. If you prefer to vary it slightly, that is fine, too, but stick with the intention, and focus on bring it to life in every aspect of your life.

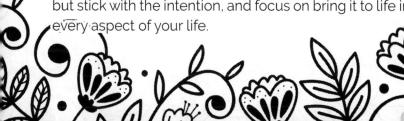

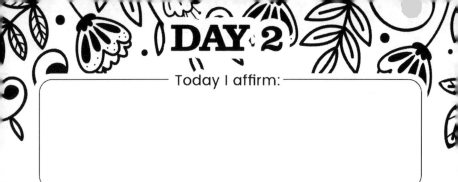

DAY 2

Today I affirm:

I want you to begin your Body Wisdom journaling with an open-ended prompt. It may seem weird or too unguided. Trust the process. You will return to this prompt several times throughout this journal. Each time you will have a different experience. Very likely, you will begin to trust yourself more and gain more information from this experience as you get more comfortable with it.

Think of a place of pain or discomfort in your body, or even a body part that you disparage.

Now, simply ask yourself, "What do I need to know or see about this?" Then allow your mind to wander.

Does it take you to another body part? Does it take you to a memory? Does it have a color or feeling associated with it? You don't need to find "the answer" – just allow your body to give you more information and insight.

Feel free to write notes about anything that comes up for you in this practice.

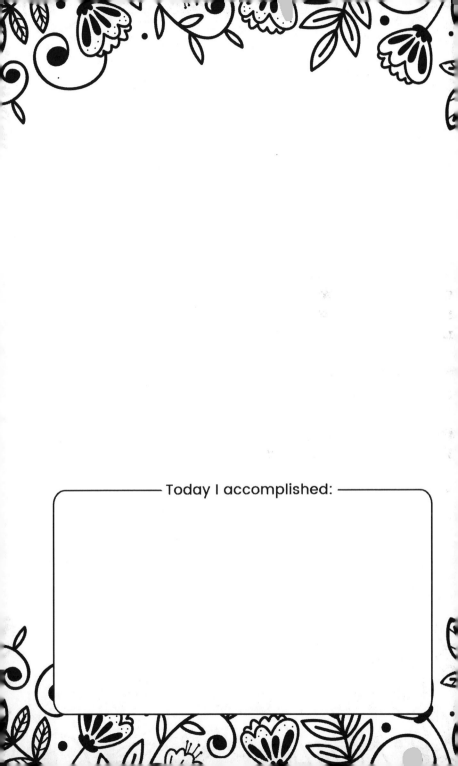

Today I accomplished:

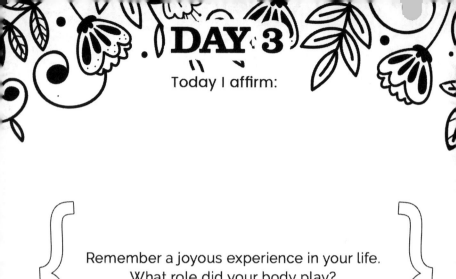

DAY 3

Today I affirm:

{ Remember a joyous experience in your life.
What role did your body play? }

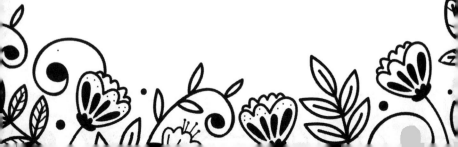

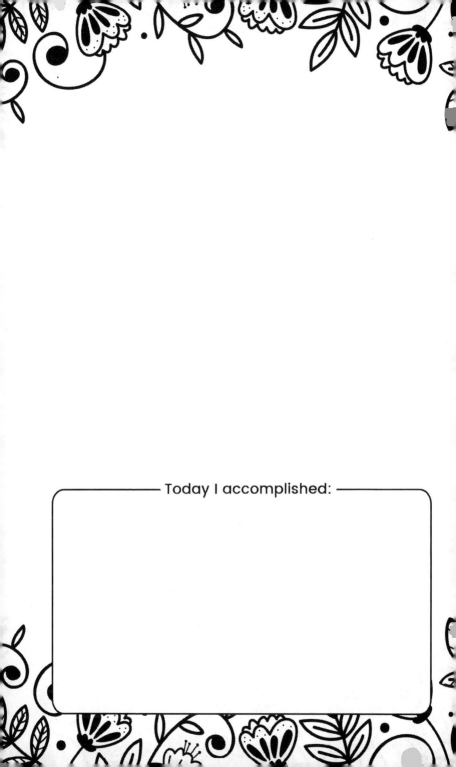

Today I accomplished:

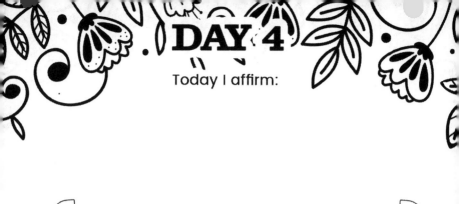

DAY 4

Today I affirm:

Think of a place in your body that is painful,
uncomfortable, tight, or you dislike.

Ask that part of your body: Where did these
negative feelings come from?

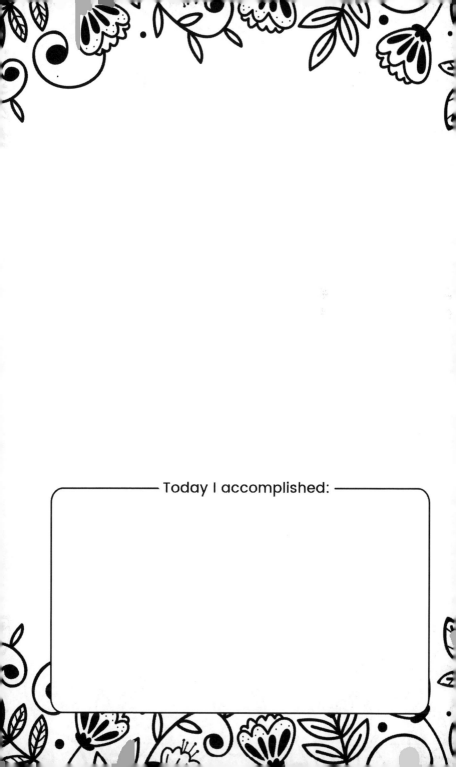

Today I accomplished:

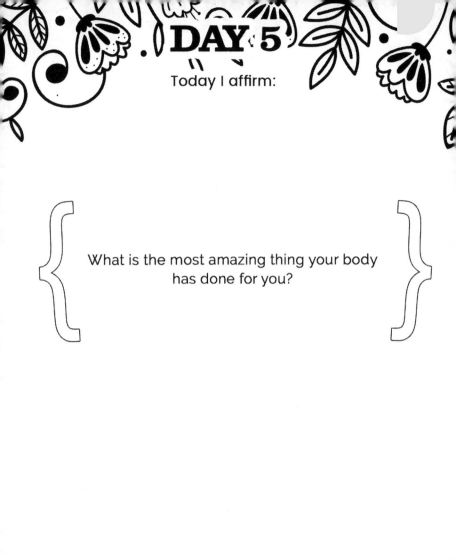

DAY 5

Today I affirm:

{ What is the most amazing thing your body has done for you? }

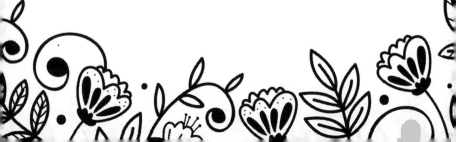

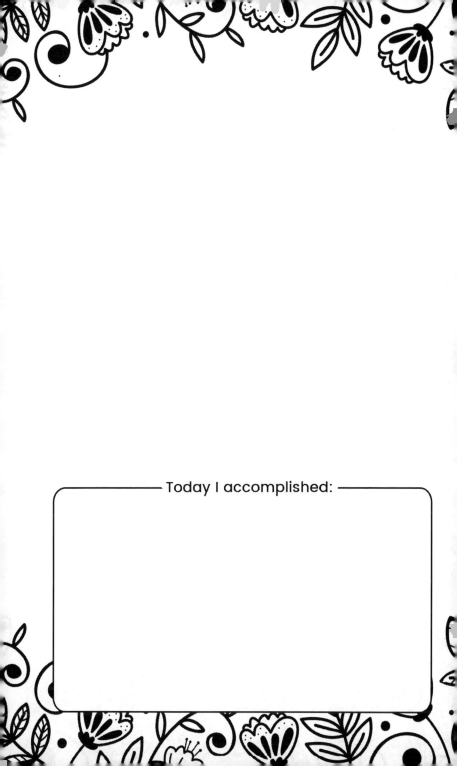

Today I accomplished:

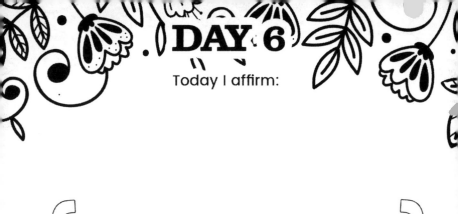

DAY 6

Today I affirm:

Think about a place in your body that has been "talking" to you lately. Ask that body part: What are you trying to tell me?

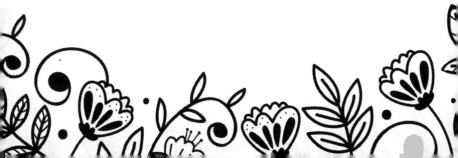

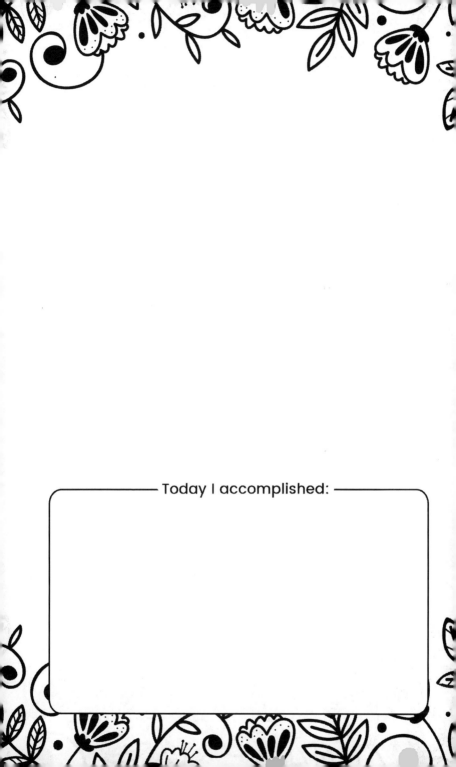

Today I accomplished:

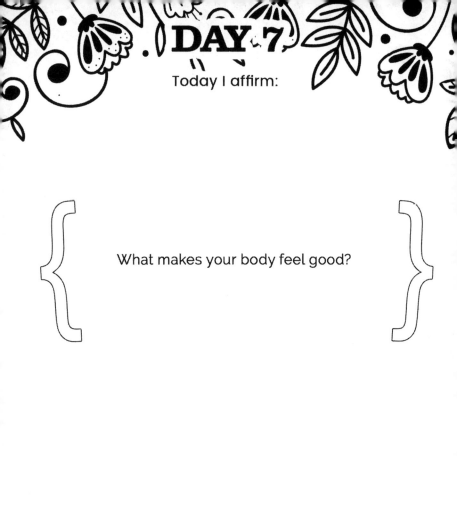

DAY 7

Today I affirm:

{ What makes your body feel good? }

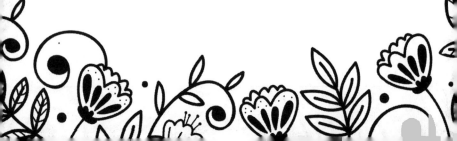

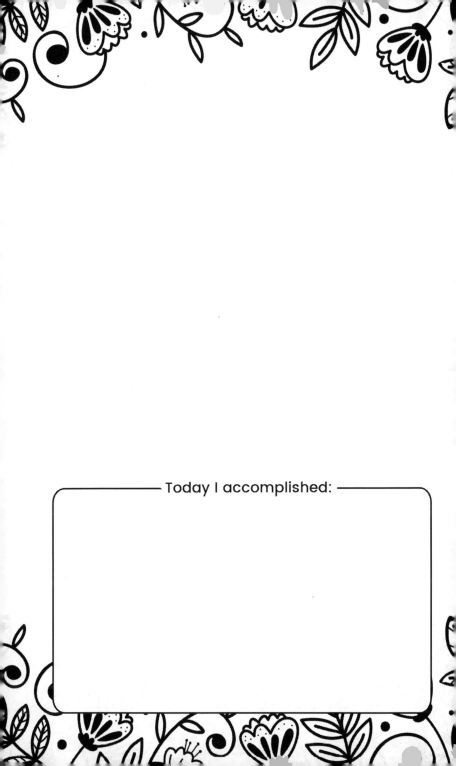

Today I accomplished:

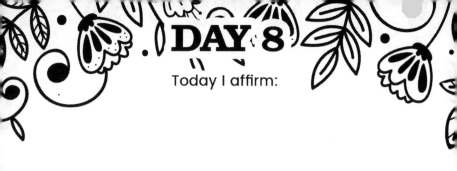

DAY 8

Today I affirm:

Think of something that you did or that happened recently that made you feel very uncomfortable. That discomfort may be affecting your body. Write about how the incident may be held in your physical body. Is there tension? Is there tightness? Is there pain?

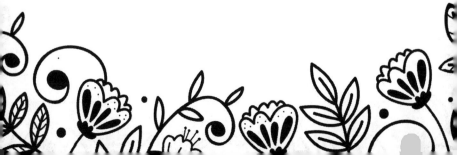

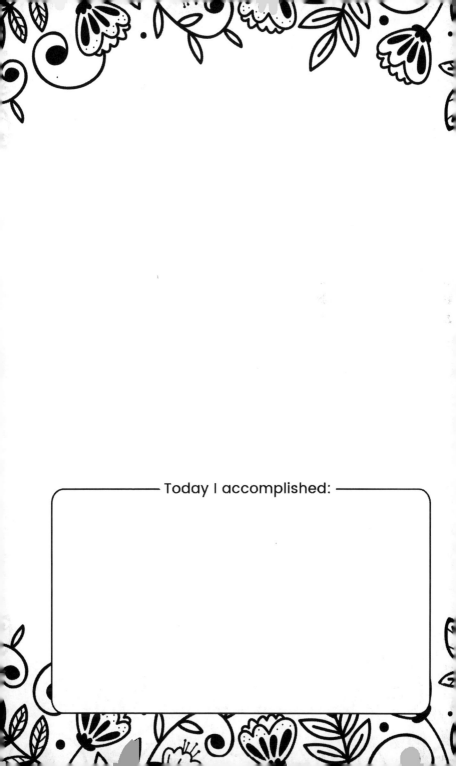

Today I accomplished:

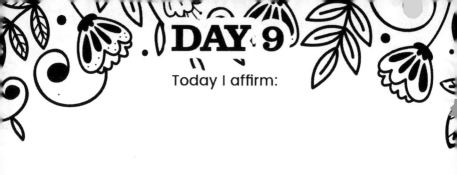

DAY 9

Today I affirm:

{ What gives you physical pleasure? This can be sensual, fun, powerful, energized, sexual, silly, strong, satisfied, or any other kind of pleasurable physical experience. }

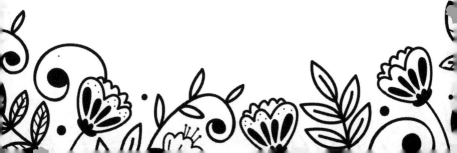

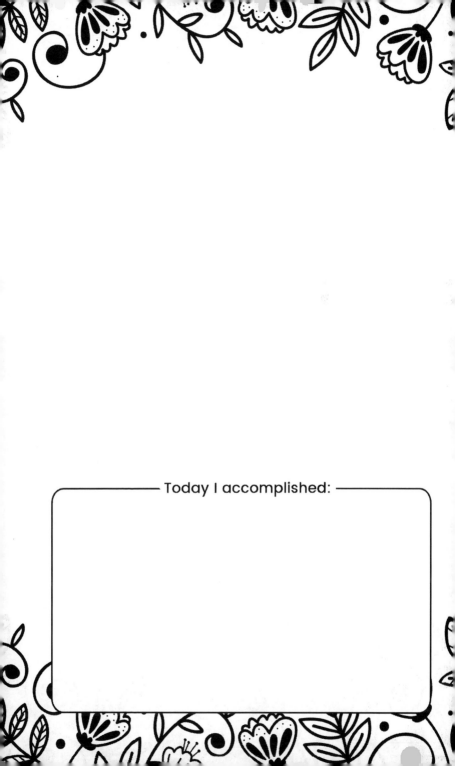

Today I accomplished:

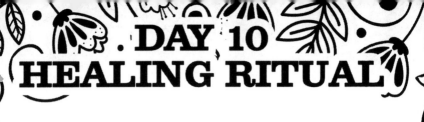

DAY 10
HEALING RITUAL

Make a list of all the things you dislike about your body. Try not to be "mean" about it... just list them out. Read through them. Acknowledge the hurt you have caused yourself by carrying this dislike. Spend some time thinking and feeling about this (5-20 minutes). When you feel you have acknowledged this completely, then it is time to move on.

Now it is time to forgive yourself. Read each line out loud as, "I forgive myself for the hurt I have caused by disliking _____. I forgive myself, and I vow to heal from this hurt. From this day forth, I will do my personal best to stop these harmful thoughts when they happen, and replace them with loving alternatives." It should take 10-30 minutes to read through each item.

Then gently pull this page out and burn it or bury it. Please do not skip this step. It is important to fully let go of the list and transform it.

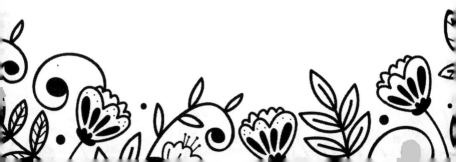

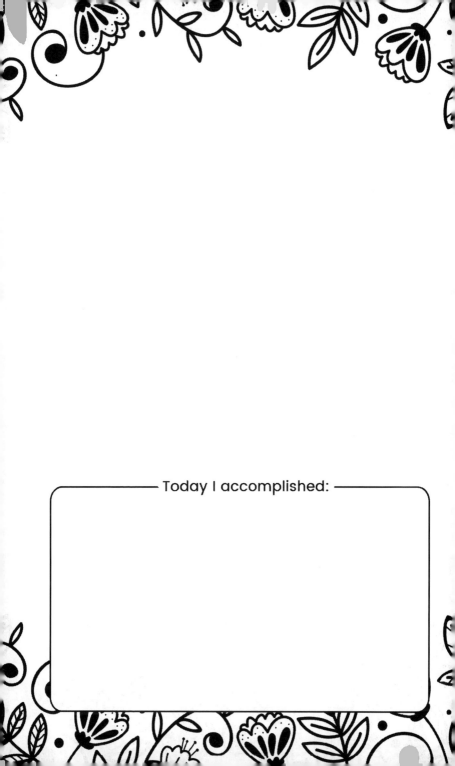

Today I accomplished:

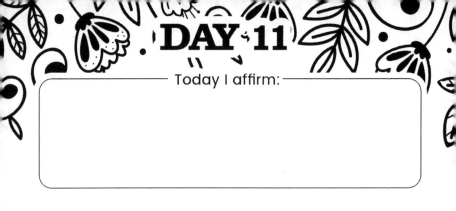

DAY 11

Today I affirm:

Let's return to the exercise in which you let your body guide you to an answer. Remember, this is truly meant to be a journey.

Try this exercise when you are feeling stressed or anxious or angry (think butterflies in stomach or feeling jittery or clenched teeth or fists). It may seem scary, as we tend to avoid stillness under stress, but it can be an empowering action.

Now, simply ask your body, "What do I need to know or see about this?" Then allow your mind to wander.

Does it take you to another body part? Does it take you to a memory? Does it have a color or feeling associated with it? You don't need to find "the answer" – just allow your body to give you more information and insight. Spend a few minutes doing this. If your mind tries to "grab" onto other thoughts, gently guide it back to the exploration.

Feel free to take notes about anything that comes up for you in this practice.

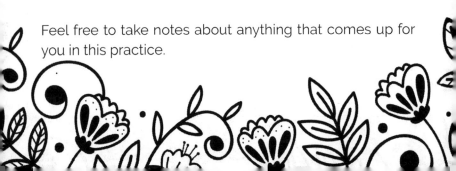

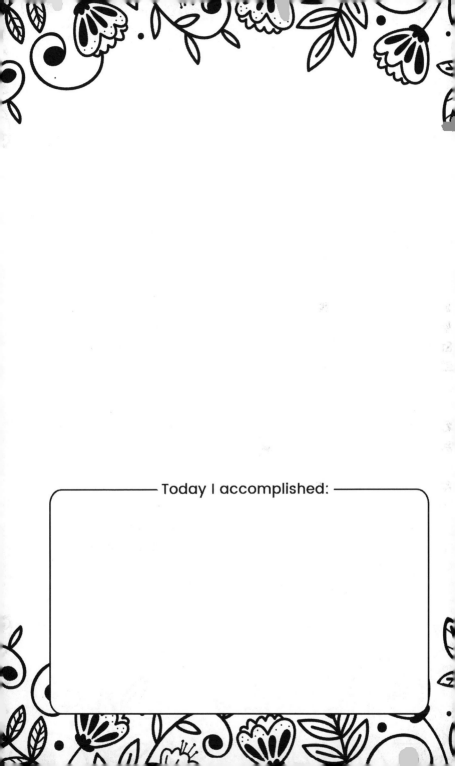

Today I accomplished:

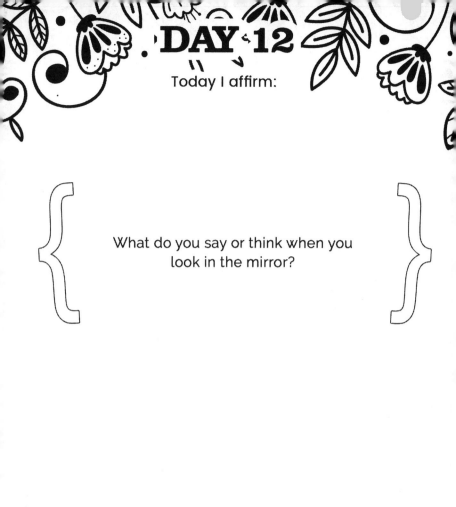

DAY 12

Today I affirm:

{ What do you say or think when you look in the mirror? }

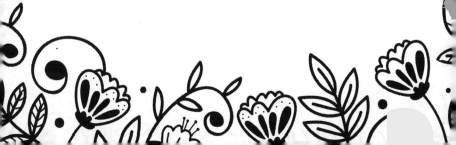

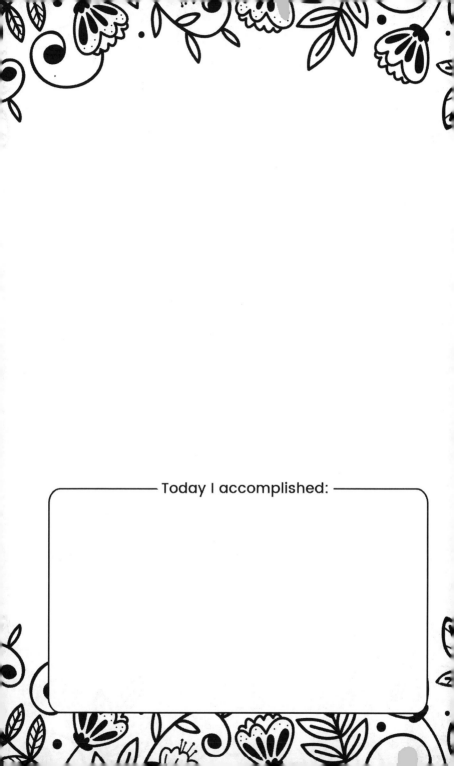

Today I accomplished:

DAY 13

Today I affirm:

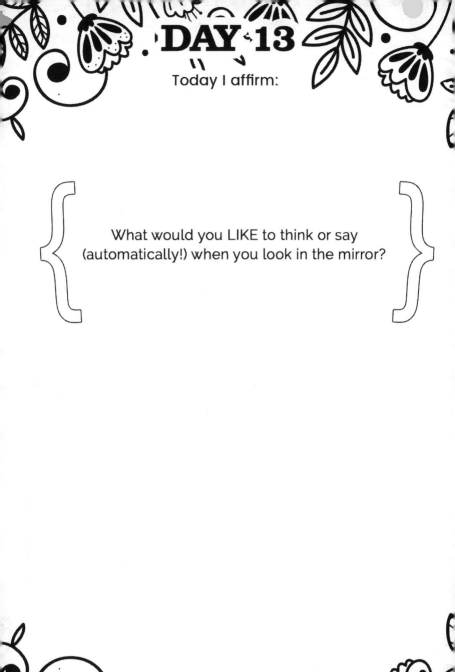

What would you LIKE to think or say
(automatically!) when you look in the mirror?

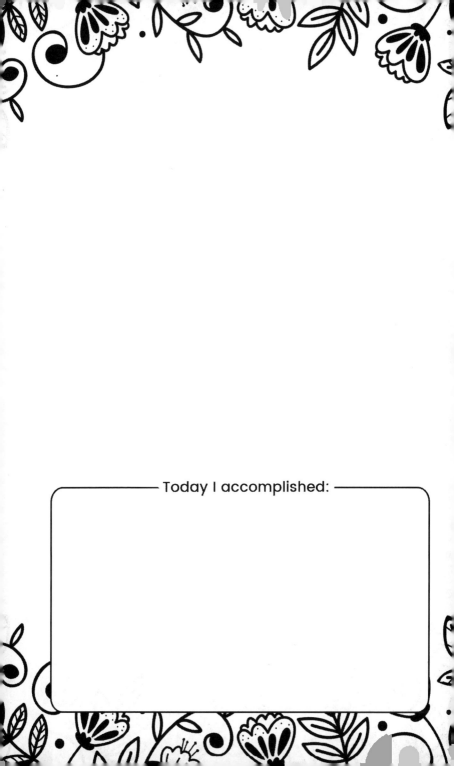

Today I accomplished:

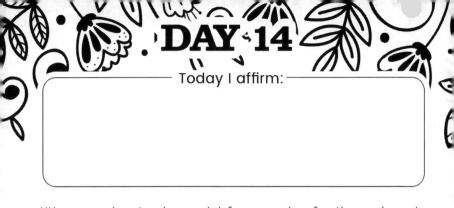

Today I affirm:

We are going to do a mini focus series for three days. I want you to go deep into the negative associations of your body, whether physical or emotional. We will spend a few days exploring the same body parts from different angles. Looking into our bodies from different perspectives helps us become more compassionate and open to insights. Sometimes the information we get isn't directly related to what we are looking at.

Think of a place in your body that is painful, uncomfortable, tight, or you dislike.

Ask yourself: How long have I felt this discomfort?

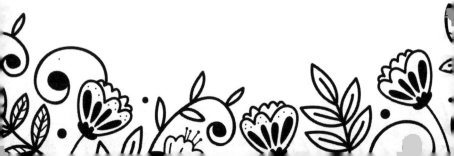

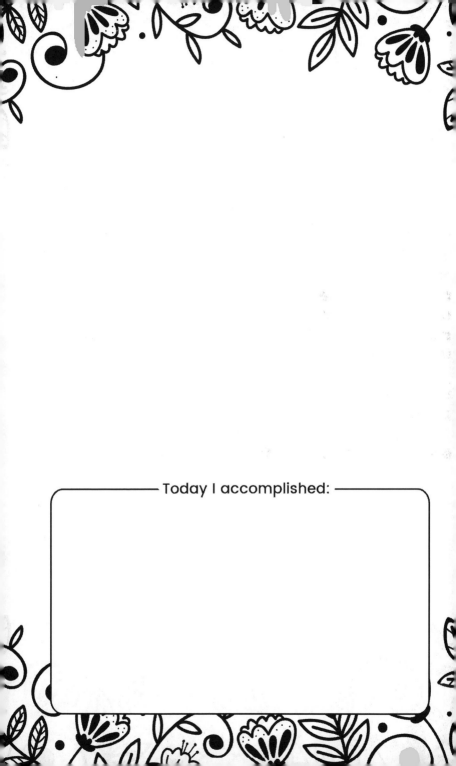

Today I accomplished:

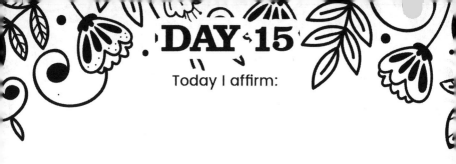

DAY 15

Today I affirm:

Think of a place in your body that is painful, uncomfortable, tight, or you dislike.

Ask that part of your body: What are you trying to teach me? If you aren't getting any answers, then ask, "How do I feel about this body part?" And always remember to let the answers flow out, even if they seem unrelated.

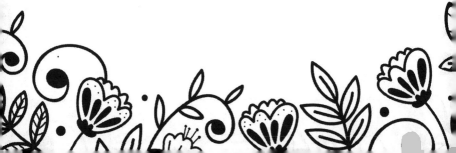

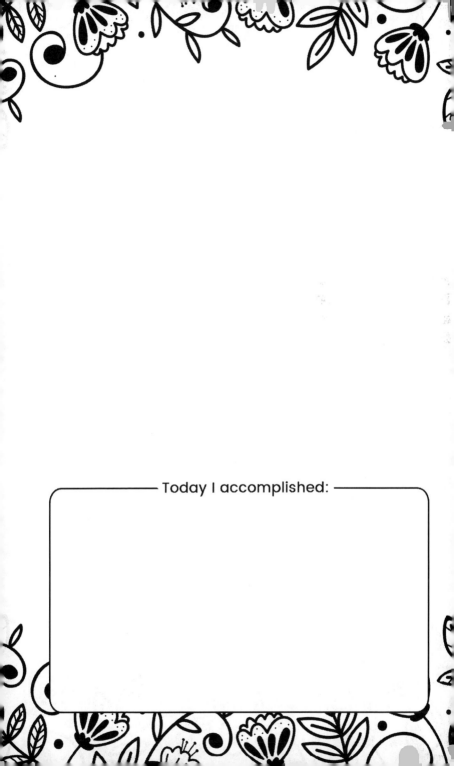

Today I accomplished:

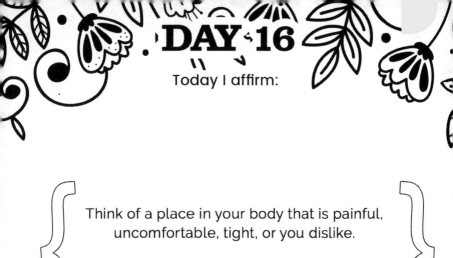

DAY 16

Today I affirm:

Think of a place in your body that is painful,
uncomfortable, tight, or you dislike.

Ask yourself: What might I need to learn from
this discomfort?

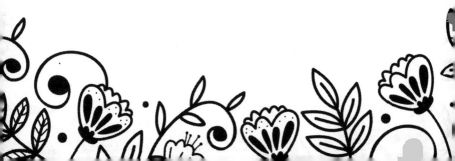

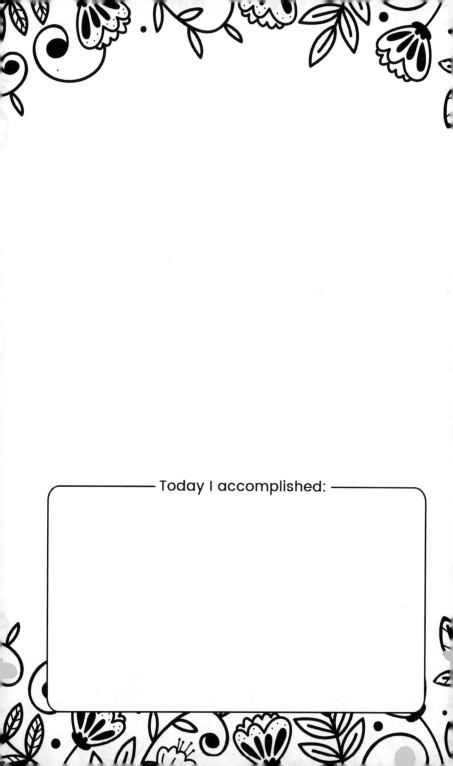

Today I accomplished:

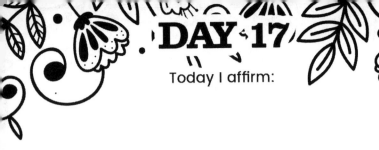

DAY 17

Today I affirm:

Do you take over the counter painkillers very often? What do you take them for? Do you know what CAUSES the pain? (Remember to think about your pain in a symbolic way, or as part of a bigger picture. What else could it mean? Refer to the dog-eared page for ideas.)

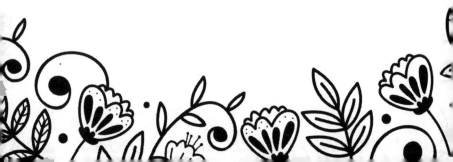

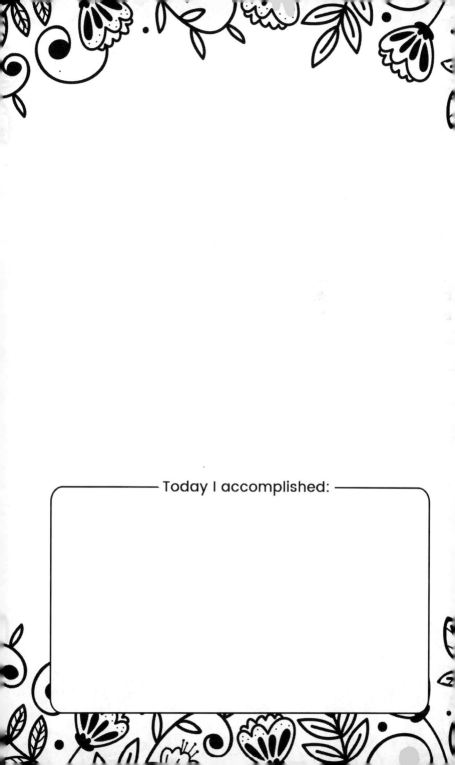

Today I accomplished:

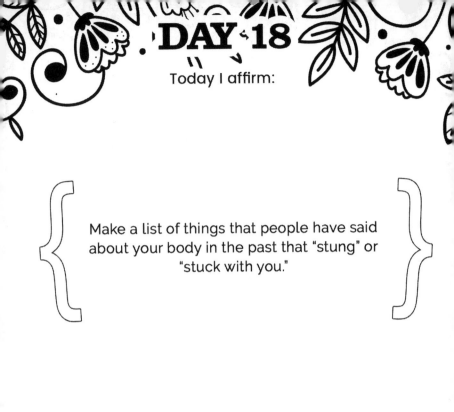

DAY 18

Today I affirm:

{ Make a list of things that people have said about your body in the past that "stung" or "stuck with you." }

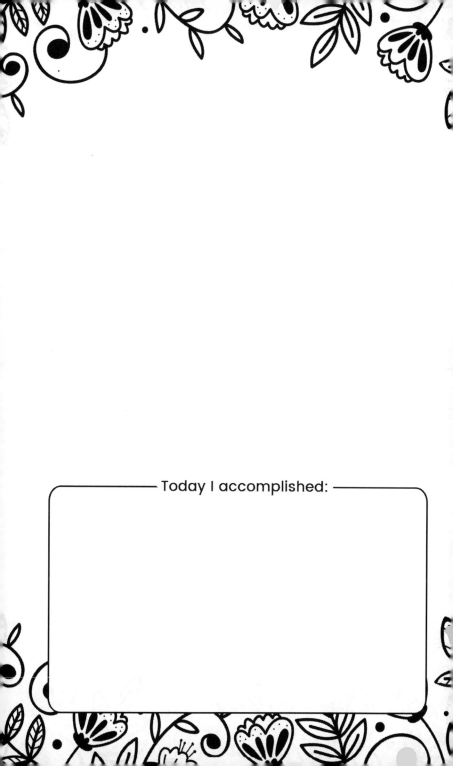

Today I accomplished:

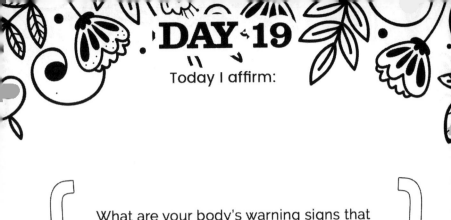

DAY 19

Today I affirm:

{ What are your body's warning signs that something is not aligned? (EX: headaches, sore muscles, lingering colds, tiredness, achy joints, poor sleep, etc.) }

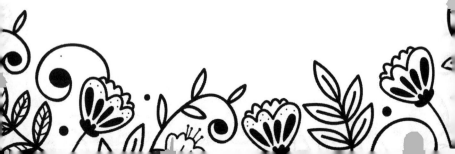

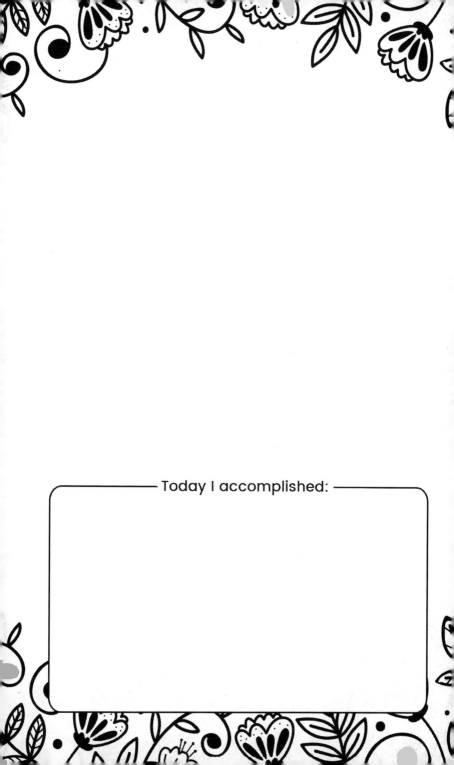

Today I accomplished:

DAY 20
HEALING RITUAL

Move through your house with an open mind. In each room, assess how many negative comments you think to yourself. You may need to do this a few times on different days. Once you identify a pattern, you should write down positive affirmations in the most triggering rooms. Put them on a pretty piece of paper or something you want to look at for a long time. Frame it if you wish.

You can boldly counter the negative self-talk you hear. For example: If you think you look old when you look in the bathroom mirror, you can write out an affirmation, "You look beautiful today!"

However, if a bold counter comment triggers a "yeah, right" reaction in your body or brain, then come at it from an angle instead. For example: If you judge your house making skills because of the pile in the laundry room, write, "You are a great listener!". This has nothing to do with the laundry, but it helps stop the cycle of judgement without causing an inner eye roll.

Helpful hint: Bathroom mirrors are a common trigger point, as are messy spots in the house (kitchen, dining table, desk). If you really want to mix things up, you can consider reducing the number of mirrors in the house, or moving their location to help reduce triggering. Place something you are proud of in its place – the wine and paint creation you did with your girlfriends, the photo of your grandma, or anything that makes you feel good.

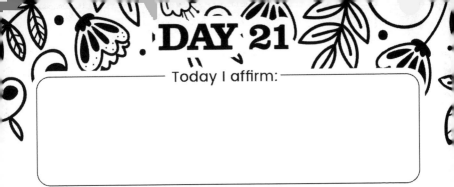

DAY 21

Today I affirm:

Think of a place in your body that you want to explore or that you feel curious about. We are starting to guide your body to share with you truthfully, as well as lovingly. There is trust between you and your body now. You are ready to hear the love it holds.

Ask yourself, "I am ready for loving truth. What can you share with me?" Then allow your mind to wander.

Does it take you to another body part? Does it take you to a memory? Does it have a color or feeling associated with it? You don't need to find "the answer" – just allow your body to give you more information and insight.

Feel free to write notes about anything that comes up for you in this practice.

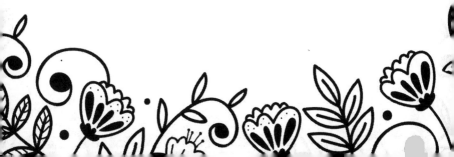

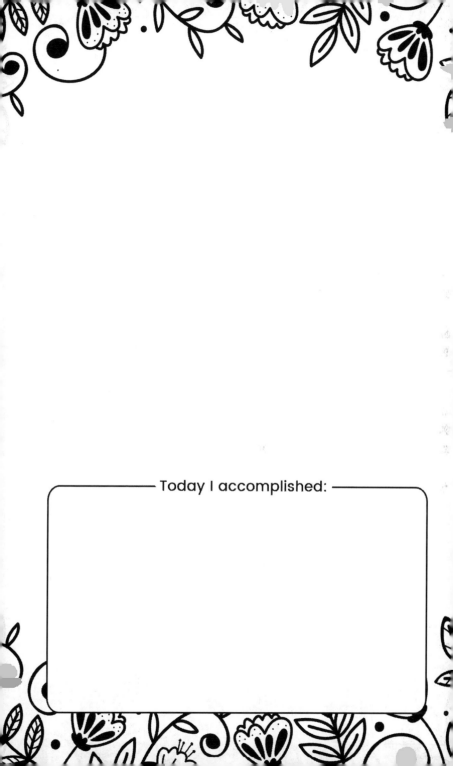

Today I accomplished:

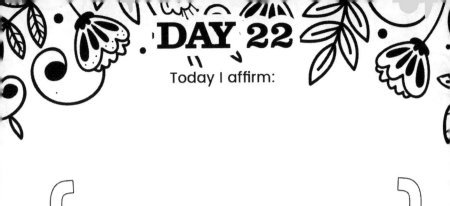

DAY 22

Today I affirm:

{ Think about a place in your body that has been "talking" to you lately. Ask that body part: What important message do you have for me? }

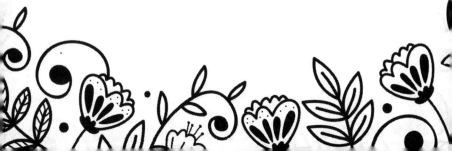

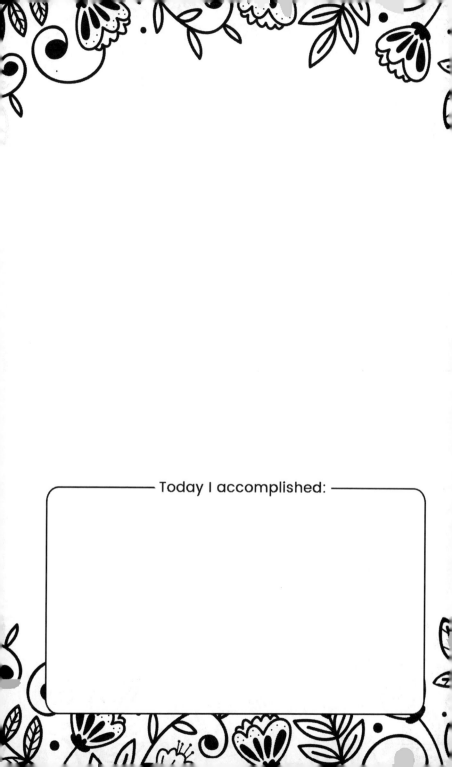

Today I accomplished:

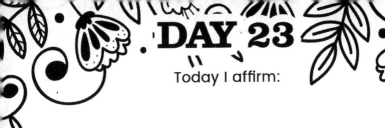

DAY 23

Today I affirm:

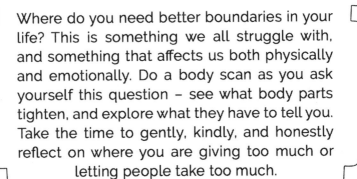

Where do you need better boundaries in your life? This is something we all struggle with, and something that affects us both physically and emotionally. Do a body scan as you ask yourself this question – see what body parts tighten, and explore what they have to tell you. Take the time to gently, kindly, and honestly reflect on where you are giving too much or letting people take too much.

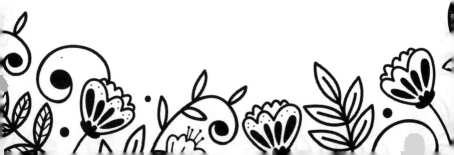

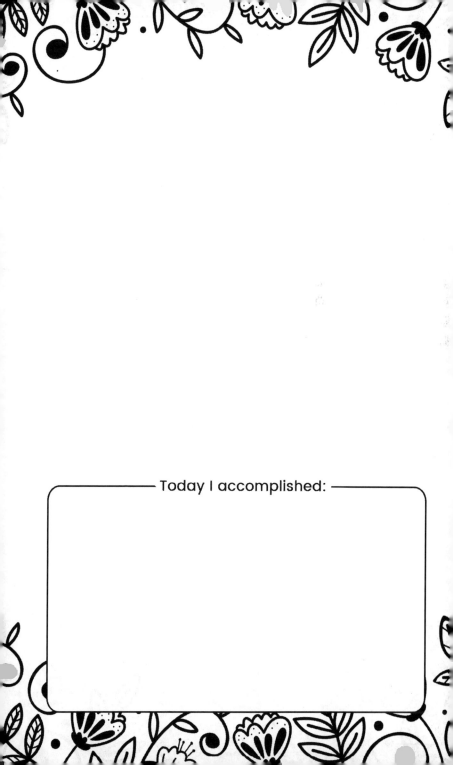

Today I accomplished:

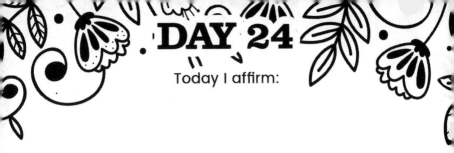

DAY 24

Today I affirm:

{
Move through your body, tuning in to what would feel good, where you could relax, and how that relates to setting boundaries that make you feel good. If it helps, brainstorm a list of simple ways to set better boundaries, such as letting a project wait until the next day and going home from work earlier. (But if that feels scary, save it for another time.)
}

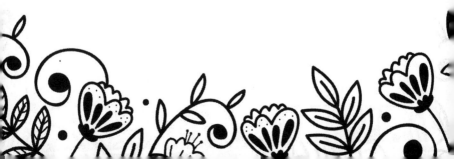

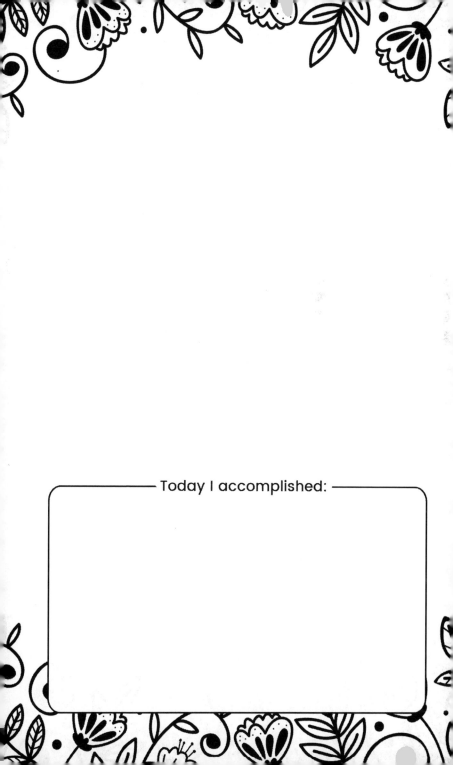

Today I accomplished:

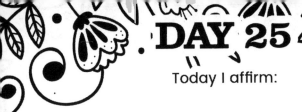

DAY 25

Today I affirm:

Think of a place where you feel like you have "an answer" for why you have pain (injury, tightness, etc.), but yet the pain is slow to resolve. Set aside the answer you usually come up with, and ask yourself: What ELSE could be the cause of this pain? (Remember to think outside the body; refer to the dog-eared page if you'd like some starting ideas.)

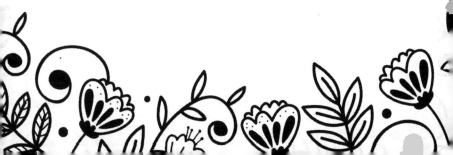

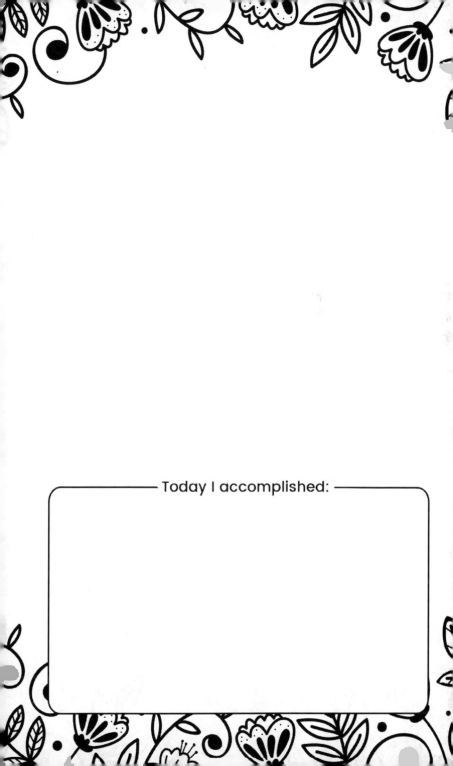

Today I accomplished:

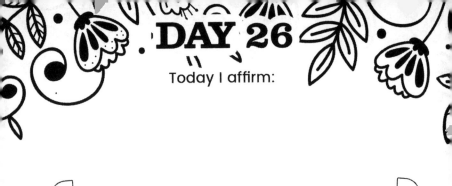

DAY 26

Today I affirm:

{
Ask your body, "What do you need?" Spend time to tune into each body part and scan for answers. Think about things that have made your body feel good in the past.
}

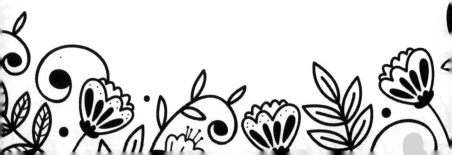

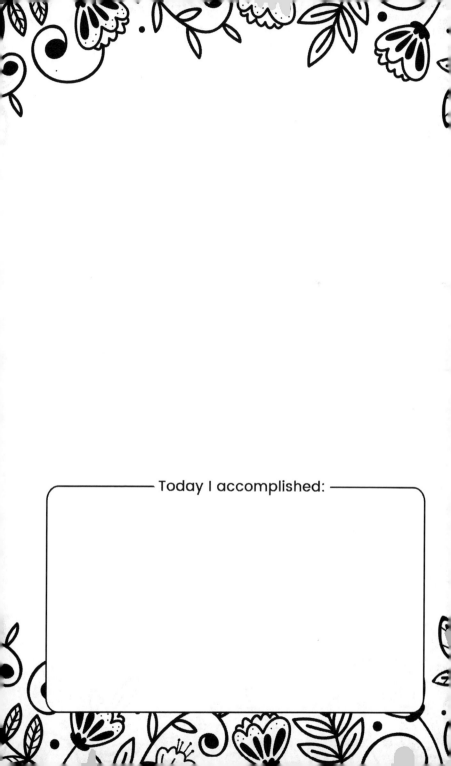

Today I accomplished:

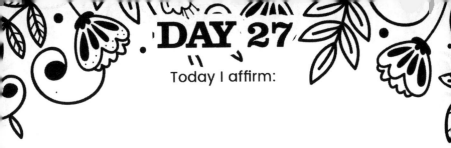

DAY 27

Today I affirm:

Brainstorm a list of activities that helps you feel strong, flexible, and joyful in your body. Dancing, running, laughing, having sex… whatever it is, put it all on this page! Consider dog-earing this page for future reference, too!

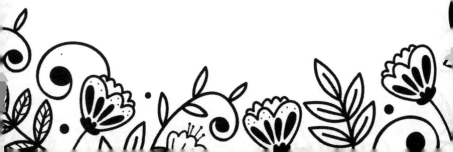

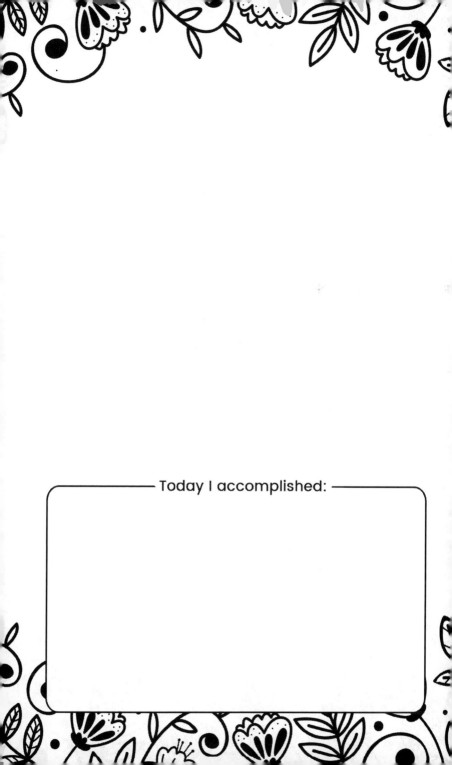

Today I accomplished:

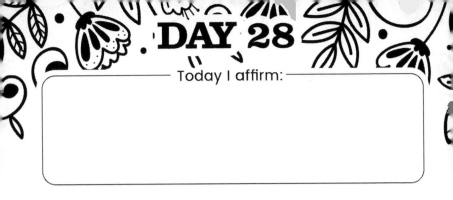

DAY 28

Today I affirm:

Think about a place with scars or wrinkles. Take a moment to consider how you can infuse those marks on your body with positive meaning. For example, wrinkles are a sign of wisdom or scars are a sign of lessons learned. Choose the meaning, and then spend a few minutes showing appreciation for those marks... thank the marks, reflect upon what you've learned from them, show some admiration or appreciation for them. Think through this slowly, with room in between for any additional thoughts that your markings share with you.

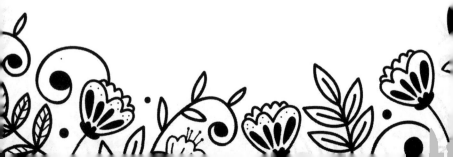

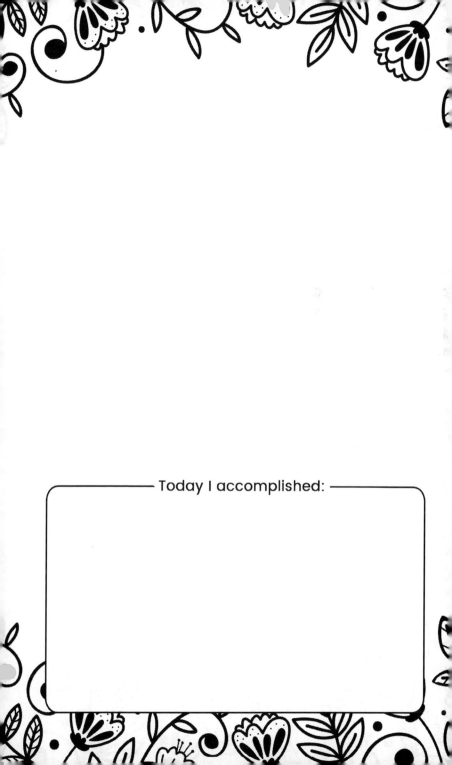

Today I accomplished:

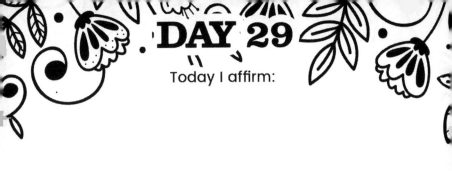

DAY 29

Today I affirm:

What foods or activities make you feel lighter, clearer, and happier?

What foods or activities make you feel heavy, bogged down, cluttered?

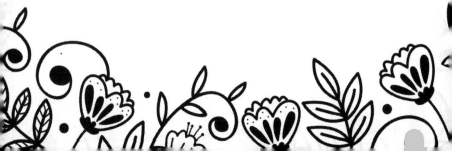

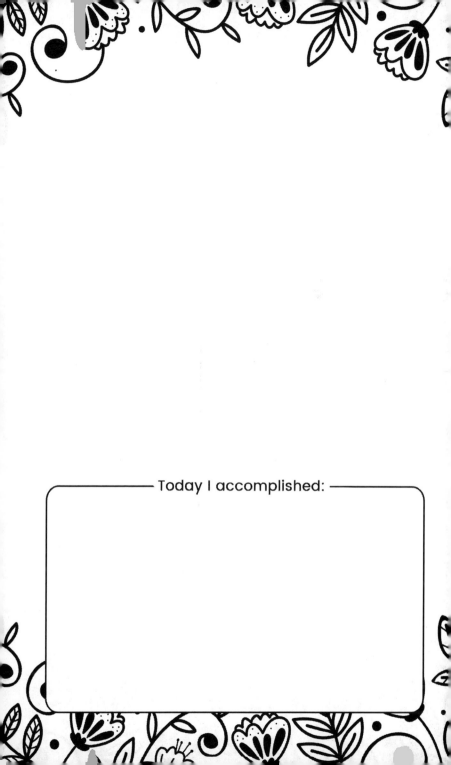

Today I accomplished:

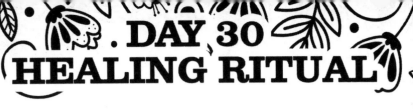

DAY 30
HEALING RITUAL

It is time to focus on the great things and great people in your life. There is nothing like digging up some powerful gratitude to change your outlook!

Spend a few minutes thinking about all the people you love and appreciate. A long lost old friend, a family member, your book club, a client or colleague, or anyone else that makes you feel good when you think about them!

Get a pack of postcards or thank you cards or beautiful note cards. Write each person a heartfelt note. It doesn't have to be complicated or overly mushy. A simple line will do the trick, "I still think about when you helped me plant that tree – thanks for being such a great friend!"

Write as many as you can! You'll walk away from this healing ritual feeling lucky in life!

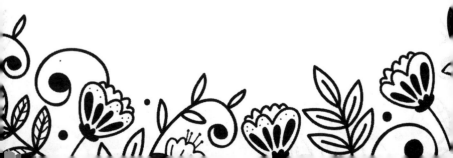

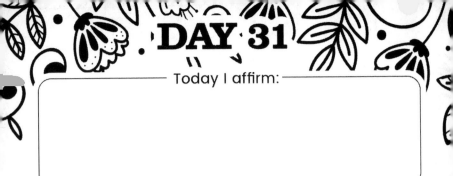

DAY 31

Today I affirm:

This is the last time I'll guide you through this particular exercise, so I want you to try it a new way. I know you're ready to start focusing on all the goodness your body holds. You have worked through a lot of the negative commentary that the outside world created for you. Now it is time to start letting your body shine!

This time, think about a body part you are starting to appreciate more, or have even come to admire or love.

Now, simply ask yourself, "What positive messages have been hiding here?" Then allow your mind to wander.

Does it take you to another body part? Does it take you to a memory? Does it have a color or feeling associated with it? You don't need to find "the answer" – just allow your body to give you more information and insight.

If you begin to feel negative messages come up, note it without judgement, and feel free to nudge yourself back to positive messaging with a thought towards your body such as, "What kind message do you have for me?"

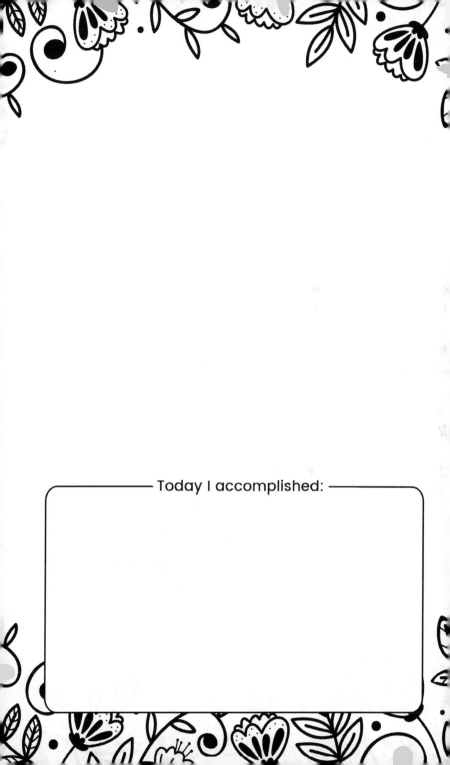

Today I accomplished:

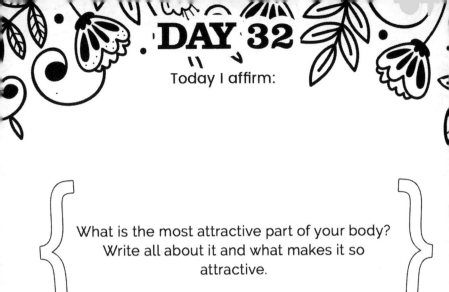

DAY 32

Today I affirm:

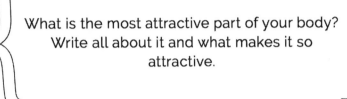

What is the most attractive part of your body?
Write all about it and what makes it so
attractive.

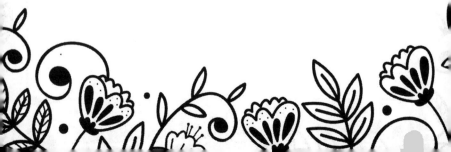

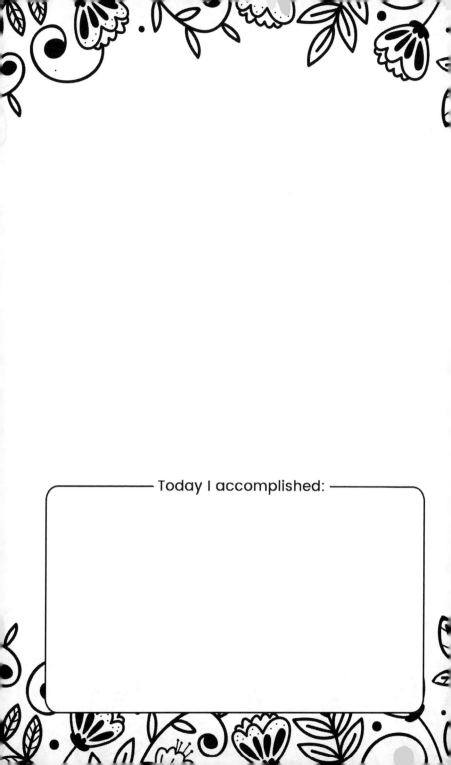

Today I accomplished:

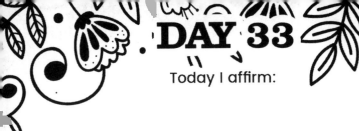

DAY 33

Today I affirm:

How can I relax my body and mind? We do not value relaxation in this crazy modern world, yet our bodies NEED it! Explore the question for higher picture feedback, or simply brainstorm a list of relaxing activities!

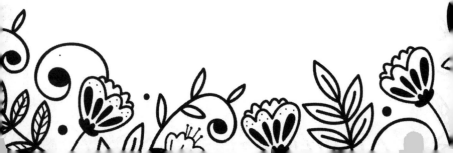

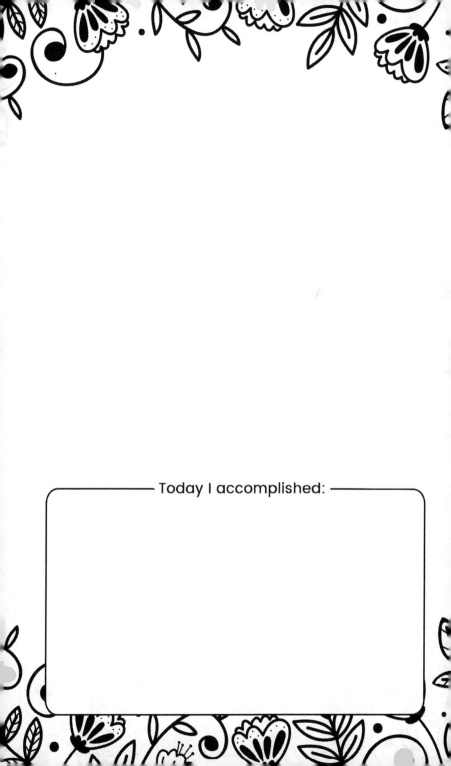

Today I accomplished:

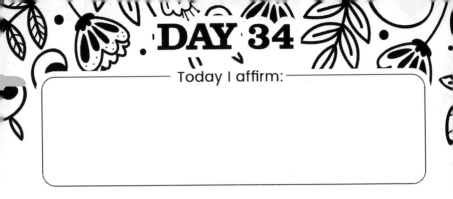

DAY 34

Today I affirm:

Get grounded today. Take off your shoes and socks, and plant your feet on the ground. Make sure the rest of your body is comfortable, however you need to sit to feel so is fine. Spend at least 5 minutes with your feet pressed into the ground. Let the ground support you and calm your nerves, mind, heart, and soul. Write out any thoughts that pop into your mind AFTER you've completed the exercise, but resist the temptation to write down all the ideas in your head WHILE doing the practice.

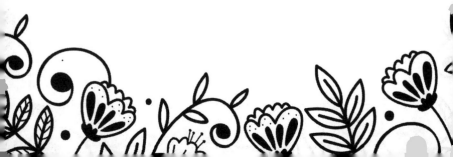

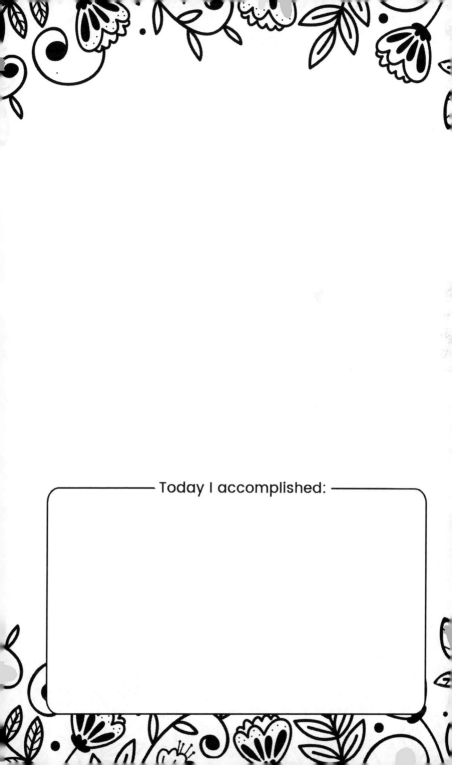

Today I accomplished:

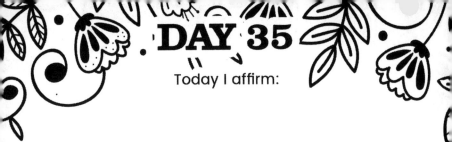

DAY 35

Today I affirm:

The next time you want to ask someone their opinion (whether in person or over the phone/text/messenger), stop and ask your body first. It doesn't matter what the question is about – the dress you are wearing, the person that annoyed you on your walk, what to make for dinner. Stop, take a deep breath, and see what your body is doing to find an answer.

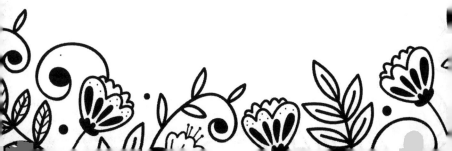

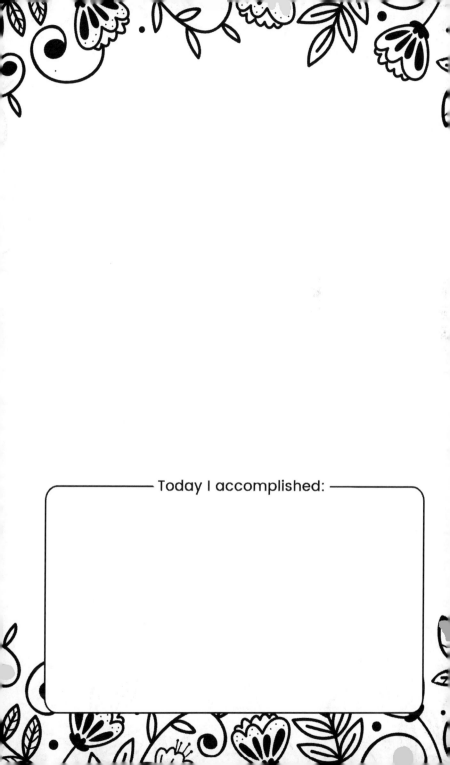

Today I accomplished:

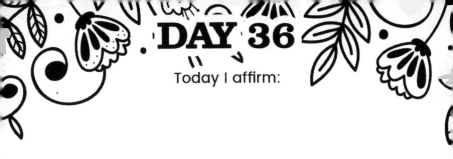

DAY 36

Today I affirm:

Was there a time you did something despite the fact that it caused you pain? This can be physical or emotional. Did you run even though your muscle was pulled? Did you sit in that workshop even though you wanted to nap? Reflect back on how you could have better listened to your body and how the outcome may have changed.

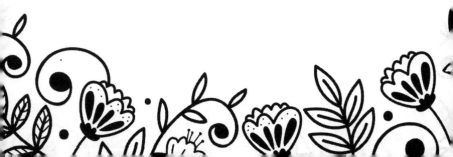

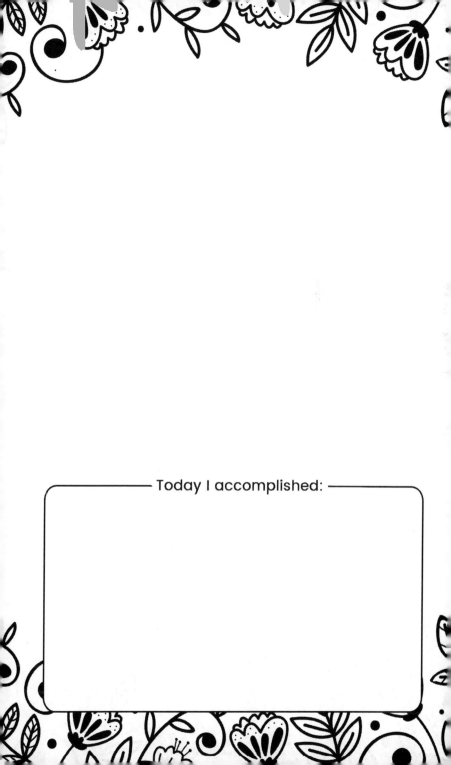

Today I accomplished:

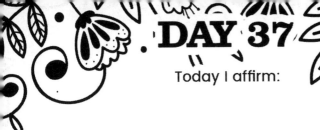

DAY 37

Today I affirm:

Just move! Sit or stand, lie down or dance. Let your body feel out the most comfortable way to be right now. Stretch, reach, swing, shake, spin... whatever it is, indulge it. Do it with music or without. Just move and trust your body's decisions. Write down any thoughts that pop into your mind AFTER you've completed the exercise, but resist the temptation to write down all the ideas in your head WHILE doing the practice.

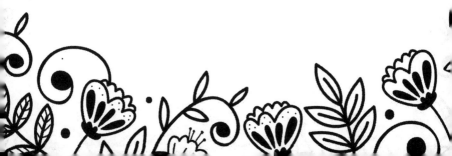

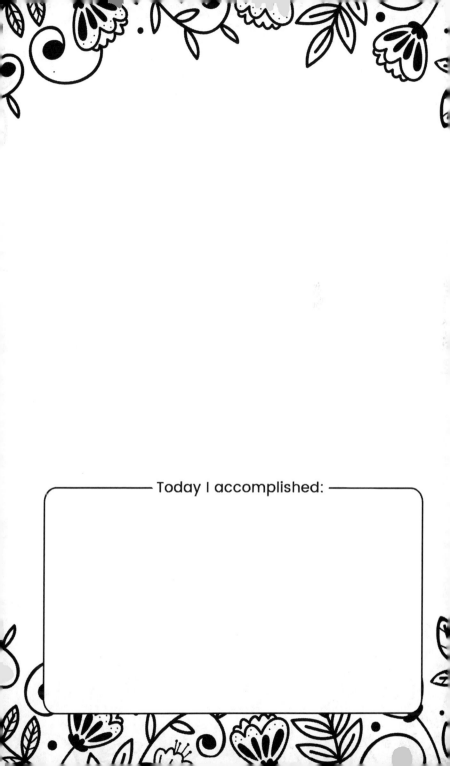

Today I accomplished:

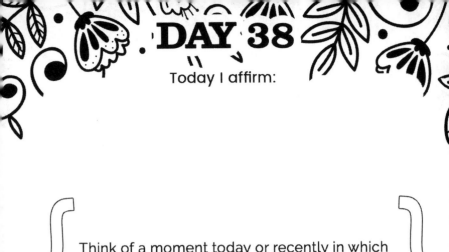

DAY 38

Today I affirm:

{ Think of a moment today or recently in which you slowed down and trusted yourself. Write about how that made you feel. }

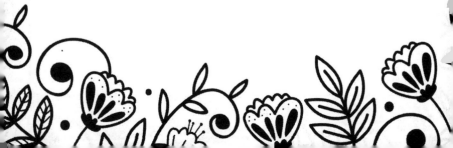

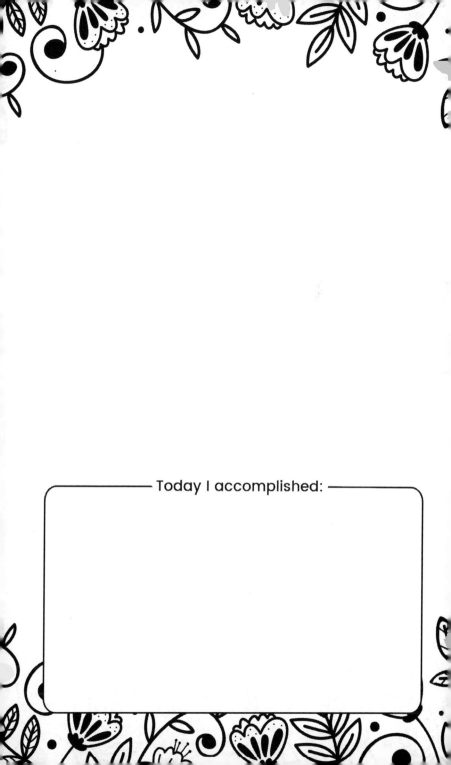

Today I accomplished:

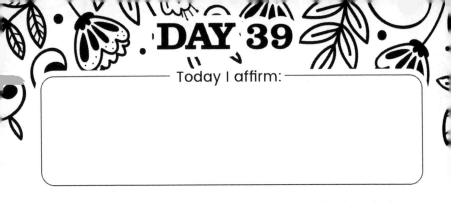

DAY 39

Today I affirm:

Spend time just breathing during your body wisdom practice today. Slow it down. Breathe deep. You can make sighing sounds if you like, or you can make it sound like wind or an ocean. Just feel that air move through your lungs, through your throat, through your mouth or nose. Feel every molecule. See what happens. It's ok if your mind runs around, just return to breathing. Do it for as long as feels just beyond comfortable. If 5 minutes sounds easy, try 10. If 30 minutes sounds easy, try 45. Let yourself release slowly. Write out thoughts that pop into your mind AFTER you've completed the exercise, but resist the temptation to write down all the ideas in your head WHILE doing the practice.

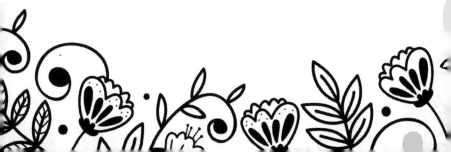

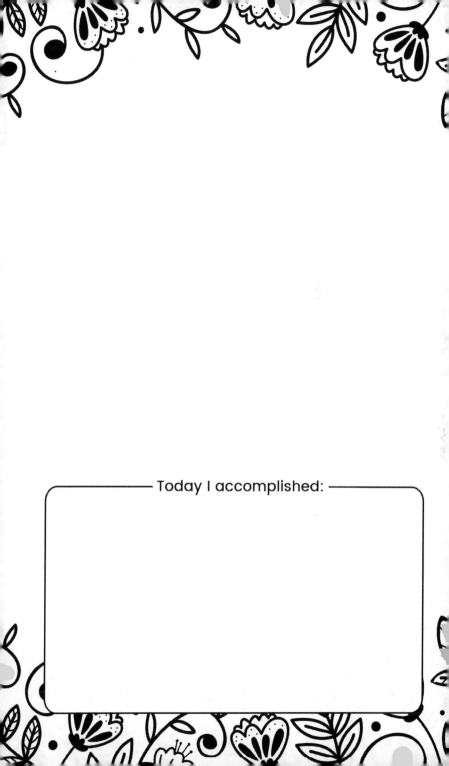

Today I accomplished:

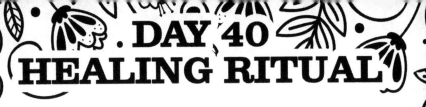

DAY 40
HEALING RITUAL

This is it... the end of the 40 days! Consider this your graduation ceremony as well as the final healing ritual. Whether it took you 40 days straight, or you did it in bits and pieces, you have done amazing personal work and healing by completing this journal.

This healing ritual can be even more powerful shared with friends at a dinner or tea party, but you can do it by yourself as well. This is your celebration of YOU.

Spend some time writing down all the positive gains you got from this journal. Write down positive thoughts you have about yourself on a regular basis. Write down a selection of affirmations from the beginning pages or elsewhere. Collect all your positive thoughts and things you've done well.

Come back to this section and refer to it when you need a pick me up! Write some of your proudest moments out and frame them, or place them in prominent places you will see often. Be proud of who you are and what you've achieved.

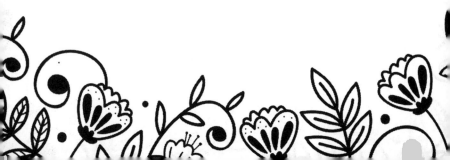

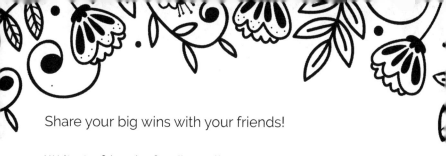

Share your big wins with your friends!

Write to friends, family, colleagues, or mentors and ask them to tell you what they appreciate or admire about you. Collect their responses in these final pages.

Write back to the friends who shared their favorite things about you, and tell them what you achieved with this journal! Let them know what you've been working on, and what you've learned, and how you've changed!

If you are doing it as an in-person celebration of you, set a date, and invite your closest friends over for tea or champagne. Ask your friends to go around and share what they love about you, or pass the journal around and have them write their thoughts in it.

Then share some of positive thoughts and achievements with your friends as part of your celebration!

The point of this final ritual is 1) to create a collection of positive thoughts about yourself from your own work, 2) to allow your loved ones to add their own words of praise and 3) to brag a little about what you've accomplished!

Have fun!

MY WINS

MY BRAGS

NEXT STEPS

Keep Journaling

If you struggle with emotional eating, stress eating, or avoidance eating... be sure to check out my other guided journal, Emotional Eating Detox: A 21-Day Inspirational Journal to Understand Your Cravings, End Overeating, and Find Freedom From Dieting Forever.

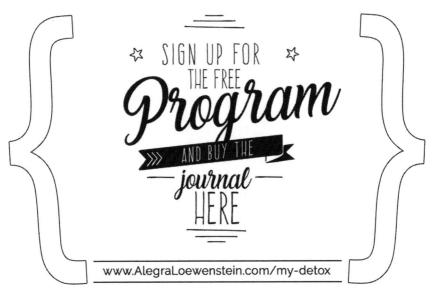

SIGN UP FOR THE FREE *Program* AND BUY THE journal HERE

www.AlegraLoewenstein.com/my-detox

This "detox" is simple. You eat whatever you want, whenever you want. You answer the journal prompts every day, and you watch a video every few days. No nonsense, no gimmicks, no protein shakes. Get to the heart of your emotional eating by being honest with yourself.

In just 5-10 minutes per day, you can discover your emotional eating triggers and your unique secret to easily overcoming them. This guided journal is designed to go beyond counting calories to allow your intuition to be your guide. You can lose weight easily, achieve your ideal weight, and eat your favorite foods without starving yourself.

If you struggle with overeating, if you find yourself craving food, if you are in binge-eating recovery, if you feel you have a food addiction, then this detox of the mind is just what you need! Get in touch with the reasons behind the struggle, so your guilt around what you eat melts away.

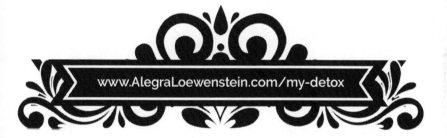

www.AlegraLoewenstein.com/my-detox

GET SUPPORT

This journal has created a strong foundation of intuition and awareness. Awareness is the most important step, but it is only the first step. You can stay stuck in awareness with no change – I stayed there for way too long, and it is my mission now to help my clients move from awareness to success as fast as possible!

Change made in isolation will never work. It's a simple fact. You might succeed for a while, but you will get sucked back into old habits. It's time to reach out to that healthy friend for lunch, to ask your family to make a healthy choice with you, and to recognize that your happiness and your health are worth investing in.

I believe in responsible financial stewardship, and I also know that every time I have invested in myself, really invested through self-care and personal development coaching, I have received benefit many times over. The same is said for my clients. It is not just worth every penny, it is actually worth so much more!

I invite you to receive one week free with my coaching app. This is my gift to you for completing this journal; it is designed to help you reclaim the sweetness in your life so you can get off the emotional eating rollercoaster (as well as the stress eating, the avoidance eating, and the bored eating!).

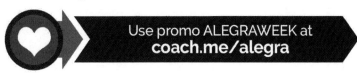

Use promo ALEGRAWEEK at
coach.me/alegra

SHARE YOUR SUCCESS

It is so important to share our goals AND our success with our community. Recently my client J.K. shared with me that she felt unsupported by her friends... until she realized that she had not actually told them what her goals were! After she did this simple thing, her perspective changed and she felt loved and uplifted by them!

So be brave. Tell a friend about this journal! Don't keep it a secret!

Tell her what you learned and how you benefited from it, and what you want to change next! We are so lucky to be able to pursue our dreams with the support of the people we love and the knowledge our society has! Yes, our society has difficult aspects, too, but we have a lot we can benefit from... and we benefit more when we take the time to share, support others, and celebrate our success! So, brag a bit about your achievements in this journal!

I would also LOVE it if you bragged to me! Let me know what you learned, how things changed, and what your biggest takeaway is!

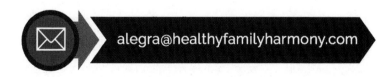

alegra@healthyfamilyharmony.com

Congratulations!

YOU HAVE SPENT 40 DAYS WORKING ON A BETTER YOU. YOU HAVE LEARNED TO TRUST YOURSELF AND YOUR BODY. KEEP UP THE AMAZING WORK!

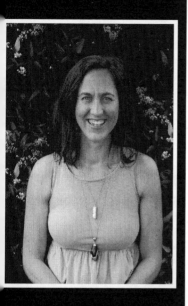

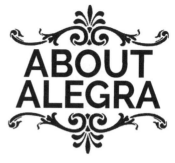

ABOUT ALEGRA

My own Body Wisdom Journey is ongoing. I've been a yogi for most of my life, but you might not know it based on how often I actually bust out a yoga mat. These days, just slowing down enough to tune in is what is most important, and I do my best to honor that.

While I have a super strong foundation of Body Wisdom, I also know how it feels to get busy and watch yourself get pushed aside and forget how to trust yourself, your

help my clients break free from the stress and worry about every thing they eat (or dreaming about what they do NOT eat).

am an avid tea drinker. drink one VERY large cup of caffeinated tea every morning (and fill it to the brim), usually black with milk. I also swear by sleepy time tea at night.

intuition, and your body. It sucks!

I also know you don't have to do anything radical to cultivate (or re-cultivate) that Wisdom. You just have to create some quiet space and listen. (Which, of course, is simple, but not necessarily easy.)

I love to help busy, high achieving women banish emotional eating so they can get off the emotional eating roller coaster and stop the yo-yo approach to health that never works! My signature program, Have Your Cake and Eat It, Too, is all about doing that in a fun, easy way without guilt, starving yourself, or swearing off your favorite foods!

Find out more at **coach.me/alegra**

Get personalized feedback on your health goals with my fun quizzes!

What Kind of Emotional Eater Are You?

www.AlegraLoewenstein.com/quiz

Which Goddess Are You?

www.AlegraLoewenstein.com/goddess

Also, while you are at it, please take a moment to share with me your biggest takeaway from this journal journey... I LOVE to hear from my readers!

alegra@healthyfamilyharmony.com

What did you learn about your body?
What changed for you?
What was the best part?

Made in the USA
San Bernardino, CA
06 June 2018